# ULTIMATE GUIDE FOR BUILDING GOOD KIDS:

# CREATING STRONG FOUNDATION FOR YOUR KIDS FUTURE SUCCESS.

**By William N. Gumm**

## **Introduction**:

Welcome to the Ultimate Guide for Building Good Kids! In this book, we will explore the many ways in which we can help our kids grow into kind, compassionate, and productive members of society. Raising kids is a challenging but rewarding experience, and with the right tools and guidance, we can ensure that our kids have the best possible start in life.

## Why Building Good Kids is Important:

As parents, we have a responsibility to help our kids develop into well-rounded individuals who are equipped to handle the challenges of life.

Building good kids is important because it helps to create a better future for us all. When kids are raised with strong values and a sense of purpose, they are more likely to succeed in school, build healthy relationships, and contribute positively to their communities.

## What You Can Expect to Learn from This Book:

In this book, we will cover a wide range of topics related to building good kids. You can expect to learn about the importance of setting boundaries, how to foster positive self-esteem, strategies for effective communication, and much more. By the end of this book, you will have a comprehensive understanding of what it takes to raise happy, healthy, and thriving children.

# TABLE OF CONTENT

# Chapter 1:

Understanding Child Development

Child development is a complex process that begins at birth and continues throughout childhood and adolescence.

Understanding the stages of child development can help parents and caregivers provide appropriate support and guidance to kids as they grow and mature.

Physical Development:
Certainly! Physical development is an important aspect of children's overall development. It involves the growth and maturation of the body, including the development of gross and fine motor skills.

Observing the characteristics of children's physical development can help parents and caregivers to identify any potential delays or issues and provide appropriate support and intervention.

It's important to provide kids with opportunities to engage in physical activities such as running, jumping, and climbing, which can help them develop their gross motor skills.

Activities such as drawing and playing with small toys can help them develop their fine motor skills.

By encouraging kids to engage in physical activities, we can help them develop a healthy body and mind. Physically active kids are more likely to be healthy and have better academic performance.

Social Development: Social development involves learning to interact with others and form relationships.

Infants begin to develop social skills by responding to their caregivers' voices and facial expressions.

As kids grow, they learn to communicate with others, share toys, and cooperate in group settings.

Certainly! Social development is a critical aspect of children's overall development.

It involves the development of social skills, such as communication, cooperation, and empathy.

Observing the characteristics of children's social development can help parents and caregivers to identify any potential issues and provide appropriate support and intervention.

It's important to provide kids with opportunities to interact with others, such as through playdates, group activities, and team sports.

By encouraging kids to engage in social activities, we can help them develop important social skills that will serve them well throughout their lives.

Socially competent kids are more likely to have positive relationships with others and be successful in school and the workplace.

Emotional Development: Certainly! Emotional development is a critical aspect of children's overall development.

It involves the development of emotional regulation, empathy, and self-awareness.

Observing the characteristics of children's emotional development can help parents and caregivers to identify any potential issues and provide appropriate support and intervention.

It's important to provide kids with opportunities to express their emotions and learn healthy ways of coping with stress and adversity.

By encouraging kids to engage in activities that promote emotional well-being, we can help them develop important emotional skills that will serve them well throughout their lives.

Emotionally competent kids are more likely to have positive relationships with others and be successful in school and the workplace.

Cognitive Development:
Certainly! Cognitive development is a critical aspect of children's overall development.

It involves the development of mental processes, such as perception, memory, language, and problem-solving.

Observing the characteristics of children's cognitive development can help parents and caregivers to identify any potential issues and provide appropriate support and intervention.

 It's important to provide kids with opportunities to learn and explore in a safe and supportive environment, which can help them develop important skills such as communication, problem-solving, and critical thinking.

By encouraging kids to engage in activities that promote cognitive development, we can help them develop important mental skills that will serve them well throughout their lives.

Kids who receive proper care and attention during their early years are more likely to grow up to be healthy, happy, and successful adults.

Factors that Influence Child Development:

Certainly! Many different factors can influence a child's development. Some of the most important factors include genetics, environment, and experiences.

Genetics refers to the traits that are inherited from parents, such as eye color or height. Environmental factors include things like nutrition, exposure to toxins, and access to healthcare.

Experiences, such as exposure to different languages or cultures, can also have a significant impact on a child's development.

Other factors that can influence child development include family dynamics, socioeconomic status, and cultural beliefs.

For example, kids who grow up in households with high levels of stress or conflict may be more likely to experience negative outcomes such as anxiety or depression.

Similarly, kids who grow up in poverty may be more likely to experience developmental delays due to a lack of access to resources such as quality healthcare and education.

Overall, it's important to recognize that many different factors can influence a child's development and that providing kids with a safe and supportive environment is essential for promoting healthy growth and development.

# Chapter 2:

Creating a Positive Home Environment

Creating a positive home environment is essential for children's well-being and development.

A positive home environment is one in which kids feel safe, loved, and supported. Here are some strategies for creating a positive home environment:

Establish Routines:

Certainly! Establishing routines for kids is an important part of promoting healthy development. Routines can help kids feel safe, secure, and in control by providing them with a sense of predictability and structure. When kids know what to expect, they are less likely to feel anxious or overwhelmed.

Routines can also help kids develop a sense of mastery and control over their environment, which can lead to increased self-confidence and self-esteem.

For example, a child who has a regular bedtime routine may feel more in control of their sleep patterns, which can lead to better sleep and improved mood. Similarly, a child who has a consistent homework routine may feel more capable and confident in their academic abilities.

Routines can help kids feel more secure and in control, which can lead to increased emotional well-being and success in all areas of life.

Additionally, Routines can help kids develop important skills such as self-regulation, time management, and responsibility by providing them with opportunities to practice these skills in a safe and supportive environment.

For example, a child who has a consistent bedtime routine may learn how to self-regulate their sleep patterns, which can help them to manage their emotions and behaviors more effectively.

Similarly, a child who has a regular homework routine may learn how to manage their time more effectively, which can help them to develop better study habits and academic skills.

Finally, a child who has a consistent routine for chores or other responsibilities may learn how to take responsibility for their actions and develop a sense of pride and accomplishment in their work.

Overall, routines can provide kids with important opportunities to develop key life skills that will serve them well throughout their lives.

Some examples of routines that can be established for kids include a regular bedtime, consistent meal times, and a daily homework schedule.

By providing kids with a predictable and structured environment, we can help them to feel more confident and capable, which can lead to increased success in school, relationships, and other areas of life—establishing routines for kids is an important part of promoting healthy development and helping kids to develop important life skills that will serve them well throughout their lives.

Encourage Open Communication: Communication is key to building strong relationships with children.

Encouraging open communication for kids helps them to feel heard, understood, and valued by creating a safe and supportive environment for them to express themselves.

When kids feel that they can talk to their parents or caregivers about their thoughts, feelings, and experiences, they are more likely to feel validated and supported. This can help to promote their overall emotional well-being and self-esteem.

Additionally, open communication can help kids develop important social and emotional skills such as empathy, active listening, and conflict resolution.

By providing kids with opportunities to practice these skills, we can help them to develop stronger relationships and a greater sense of connection with others.

they were encouraging open communication with kids, an important part of promoting their emotional well-being, social development, and overall happiness.

When kids feel that they can talk to their parents or caregivers about their thoughts, feelings, and experiences, they are more likely to develop positive relationships and a strong sense of self-worth.

Additionally, Open communication helps kids develop important social and emotional skills such as empathy, active listening, and conflict resolution by providing them with opportunities to practice these skills in a safe and supportive environment.

When kids feel that they can talk to their parents or caregivers about their thoughts, feelings, and experiences, they are more likely to develop a greater sense of empathy and understanding toward others.

This can help them to develop stronger relationships and a greater sense of connection with others.

Additionally, open communication can help kids develop active listening skills, which are essential for effective communication and interpersonal relationships.

Finally, open communication can help kids develop conflict-resolution skills, which are essential for navigating social situations and resolving interpersonal conflicts.

By providing kids with opportunities to practice these skills, we can help them to develop stronger social and emotional skills that will serve them well throughout their lives.

Some ways to encourage open communication with kids include actively listening to what they have to say, asking open-ended questions, and responding with empathy and understanding.

By creating a safe and supportive environment for kids to express themselves, we can help them to develop important life skills and promote their overall well-being.

Set Clear Boundaries: Setting clear rules and consequences for behavior can help kids understand what is expected of them and feel more in control.

Setting clear boundaries is important for creating a positive home environment because it helps to promote a sense of safety, security, and predictability for everyone involved.

When parents or caregivers set clear boundaries for children, it helps to establish expectations and guidelines for behavior, which can help to reduce conflict, confusion, and stress.

Kids who understand the rules and expectations of their home environment are more likely to feel safe and secure, as they know what to expect and what is expected of them.

This can help to reduce anxiety and promote a sense of stability and predictability.

Additionally, Clear boundaries can help to promote a sense of trust and respect between family members, as everyone learns to understand and respect each other's needs, wants, and boundaries.

When family members understand and respect each other's boundaries, it helps to create a safe and supportive environment where everyone feels heard, valued, and respected.

This can help to promote healthy communication and positive relationships between family members, which can have a positive impact on everyone's mental and emotional well-being.

By setting clear boundaries and expectations, parents or caregivers can help to create a positive home environment where everyone feels safe, supported, and valued.

By setting clear boundaries, parents or caregivers can create a positive home environment that promotes healthy communication, mutual respect, and positive relationships between family members.

When parents or caregivers set clear boundaries for children, it helps to establish expectations and guidelines for behavior, which can help to reduce conflict, confusion, and stress.

Additionally, Clear boundaries can help to promote a sense of responsibility and accountability as kids learn to understand the consequences of their actions and how to make positive choices that align with family values and expectations.

When parents or caregivers set clear boundaries for children, they establish expectations and guidelines for behavior, which can help kids understand what is expected of them.

By doing this, kids learn that their actions have consequences, which can help them to develop a sense of responsibility and accountability for their behavior.

When the kid understands the consequences of their actions, they are more likely to make positive choices that align with family values and expectations.

For example, if a child knows that they are expected to complete their homework before watching TV, they are more likely to prioritize their homework and make positive choices that align with this expectation.

This can help kids develop a sense of responsibility and accountability, which can have a positive impact on their overall development and well-being.

In addition, clear boundaries can help kids develop a sense of self-discipline and self-control as they learn to regulate their behavior according to established guidelines. This can help kids develop important life skills that will serve them well throughout their lives.

By setting clear boundaries, parents or caregivers can help kids develop a sense of responsibility, accountability, and self-discipline, which can have a positive impact on their overall development and well-being.

Finally, clear boundaries can help to promote a sense of respect and mutual understanding between family members, as everyone learns to understand and respect each other's needs, wants, and boundaries.

By setting clear boundaries, parents or caregivers can create a positive home environment that promotes healthy communication, mutual respect, and positive relationships between family members.

Spend Quality Time Together: Spending quality time with your kids is essential for building strong relationships because it helps to create a sense of connection and trust between family members.

When parents or caregivers spend quality time with their children, they show that they value and care about their children, which can help to build a positive and supportive relationship.

Quality time can take many forms, such as playing games, reading books, going for walks, or simply talking and listening to each other.

By spending time together, parents or caregivers can learn more about their children's interests, concerns, and needs, which can help to build a deeper understanding and connection between family members.

In addition, spending quality time with kids can help to create positive memories and experiences that kids will remember for years to come.

These positive memories can help to build a sense of security and trust, which can have a positive impact on children's overall development and well-being.

Finally, spending quality time with kids can also help to promote healthy communication and positive relationships between family members.

By spending time together, parents or caregivers can model positive communication skills and help kids develop important social and emotional skills.

This can help to create a positive and supportive family environment where everyone feels valued, heard, and respected.

# Chapter 3:

Teaching Values and Behaviors

Teaching values and behaviors is an important part of raising a good kid.

By instilling positive values and behaviors, parents or caregivers can help kids develop important life skills and become responsible, caring, and compassionate individuals.

In this chapter, we will explore some strategies for teaching values and behaviors to children.

Identifying Core Values

Before you can teach values and behaviors to your children, it's important to identify your core values.

What do you believe in? What values are important to you? Some common values include honesty, kindness, respect, responsibility, and compassion.

By identifying your core values, you can model these values for your kid and help them to understand why they are important.

Strategies for Teaching Values and Behaviors

There are many strategies that parents or caregivers can use to teach values and behaviors to children. Here are a few examples:

1. Lead by example: kids learn through observation and imitation, especially in their early years.

They learn by watching the people around them, including their parents or caregivers, and modeling their behavior.

kids are like sponges, soaking up everything they see and hear. They are constantly learning from their environment and the people in it.

When parents or caregivers model positive behaviors, kids are more likely to imitate those behaviors.

For example, if a child sees their parent being kind and respectful to others, they are more likely to exhibit those same behaviors.

Conversely, if a child sees their parent being rude or aggressive, they may imitate those negative behaviors.

Therefore, parents or caregivers need to model the behaviors they want their kids to exhibit.

2. Use positive reinforcement: Positive reinforcement is a powerful tool for teaching values and behaviors to kids because it rewards positive behavior and encourages kids to continue exhibiting that behavior.

Positive reinforcement can take many forms, such as praise, rewards, or privileges. When a child exhibits positive behavior, such as being honest or showing kindness, parents or caregivers can use positive reinforcement to encourage the child to continue exhibiting that behavior.

For example, if a child shares their toys with a sibling, the parent can praise the child and offer a reward, such as extra playtime or a special treat.

This positive reinforcement can help the child understand that sharing is a positive behavior and encourage them to continue sharing in the future.

Positive reinforcement can also help kids develop a positive self-image and boost their self-esteem.

When kids are praised and rewarded for positive behavior, they feel good about themselves and are more likely to exhibit positive behavior in the future.

This positive cycle can help kids develop positive values and behaviors that will serve them well throughout their lives.

positive reinforcement is a powerful tool for teaching values and behaviors to kids because it rewards positive behavior, encourages kids to continue exhibiting that behavior, and helps them develop a positive self-image and boost their self-esteem.

3. Use consequences: Consequences can be an effective tool for teaching values and behaviors to kids because they help kids

understand that their actions have consequences.

When kids exhibit negative behavior, such as lying or being disrespectful, parents or caregivers can use consequences to help the child understand that their behavior is not acceptable.

Consequences can take many forms, such as loss of privileges, time-outs, or natural consequences. For example, if a child is caught lying, the parent can explain that lying is not acceptable and that there will be consequences for their actions, such as loss of screen time or a time-out.

This consequence helps the child understand that their behavior has consequences and encourages them to exhibit positive behavior in the future.

Consequences can also help kids develop empathy and understanding for others.

Consequences can help kids develop empathy and understanding for others because they provide an opportunity for kids to reflect on their behavior and the impact it has on others.

When their kids experience consequences for their negative behavior, they can develop a better understanding of how their actions affect others and how they can make amends for their behavior.

For example, if a child is caught lying, the parent can explain how their behavior has hurt others and the importance of being honest. The child may be required to apologize to the person they lied to and make amends for their behavior.

Developed this experience can help the child empathy and understanding for others by helping them understand the impact of their actions on others and the importance of making things right.

Consequences can also help kids develop problem-solving skills and learn from their mistakes. When their kid experience consequences for their negative behavior, they can reflect on what they did wrong and how they can do better in the future. This can help kids develop positive values and behaviors, such as honesty and respect.

Consequences can help kids develop empathy and understanding for others by providing an opportunity for reflection and making amends for negative behavior.

This experience can help kids develop problem-solving skills and learn from their mistakes, which can help them develop positive values and behaviors that will serve them well throughout their lives.

Consequences can be an effective tool for teaching values and behaviors to kids because they help kids understand that their actions have consequences, encourage them to exhibit positive behavior in the future, and help them develop empathy and understanding for others.

4. Use teachable moments: Teachable moments help teach kids about values and behaviors because they provide an opportunity for kids to learn in real-life situations

Teachable moments are unplanned opportunities that arise naturally during everyday life.

These moments can provide valuable opportunities for parents or caregivers to teach kids about values and behaviors in a way that is meaningful and relevant to their lives.

For example, if a child sees a homeless person on the street, this can be a teachable moment for parents or caregivers to talk to the child about empathy, kindness, and the importance of helping others.

This real-life situation can help the child understand the importance of treating others with kindness and compassion.

Teachable moments can also help kids develop critical thinking skills and learn to make good decisions.

When their kid encounters real-life situations, they have an opportunity to think through the situation and make decisions based on their values and beliefs.

This can help kids develop positive values and behaviors, such as honesty and responsibility.

Teachable moments help teach kids about values and behaviors because they provide an opportunity for kids to learn in real-life situations.

These moments can help kids develop critical thinking skills, learn to make good decisions, and develop positive values and behaviors that will serve them well throughout their lives.

Modeling Good Behavior
Modeling good behavior is one of the most important strategies for teaching values and behaviors to kids because kids learn by example.

When parents or caregivers model good behavior, they provide a powerful example for kids to follow.

Kids who see adults behaving positively and respectfully are more likely to develop positive values and behaviors themselves.

# Chapter 4:

Encouraging Learning and Growth
Education and learning are critical for children's development and future success.

Encouraging learning and growth is an essential part of building good kids. In this chapter, we will discuss the importance of education and learning, strategies for encouraging learning and growth, and building resilience and a growth mindset.

The Importance of Education and Learning

Education and learning are essential for children's development. Education provides kids with the knowledge and skills they need to succeed in life.

Learning helps kids develop critical thinking skills, problem-solving abilities, and creativity. Education and learning also help kids build self-esteem and confidence.

Strategies for Encouraging Learning and Growth

There are many strategies parents can use to encourage learning and growth in their children.

One of the most effective strategies is to create a positive learning environment; Parents create a positive learning environment for their kids by providing a space that is conducive to learning.

This means creating a quiet and comfortable space where kids can study, read, and learn without distractions.

Parents can also provide kids with the tools they need to learn, such as books, educational toys, and technology.

In addition to the physical environment, parents can create a positive learning environment by setting aside time each day for homework and reading.

This helps kids develop good study habits and encourages them to take learning seriously.

Parents can also encourage kids to ask questions and explore their interests, which helps kids develop a love of learning.

Encouraging kids to ask questions and explore their interests is important because it helps kids develop a love of learning.

When kids are interested in a topic, they are more likely to engage with it and learn more about it. This can lead to a lifelong love of learning and a desire to explore new topics and ideas.

Parents can encourage kids to ask questions and explore their interests by providing opportunities for learning and exploration.

This can include things like taking kids to museums, libraries, and other educational spaces, providing books and other resources on topics that interest them, and engaging in conversations about their interests.

Encouraging kids to ask questions and explore their interests also helps kids develop critical thinking skills. When kids are encouraged to ask questions and explore their interests, they learn how to think critically about the world around them and develop problem-solving skills. This can help them succeed in school, work, and life in general.

Creating a positive learning environment also involves providing emotional support and encouragement to children. Parents can praise their kids for their efforts and progress rather than just their achievements.

This helps kids develop self-esteem and confidence, which in turn helps them take on new challenges and persevere through difficult tasks.

Creating a positive learning environment is essential for children's development. It helps kids develop a love of learning and provides them with the tools and support they need to succeed in life.

Another strategy for encouraging learning and growth is to provide kids with opportunities to learn outside of the classroom. Encouraging learning and growth is important because it helps kids develop critical thinking skills, problem-solving abilities, and creativity.

Learning outside of the classroom provides kids with opportunities to explore their interests and learn about the world around them in a hands-on way.

When kids are exposed to new experiences and ideas, they are more likely to develop a love of learning. This can help them become lifelong learners and pursue their passions throughout their lives.

Encouraging learning and growth by providing kids with opportunities to learn outside of the classroom is essential for children's development. It helps them become well-rounded individuals who are prepared to succeed in life.

Building Resilience and a Growth Mindset

They were building resilience, and a growth mindset for kids is important because it helps them develop the skills they need to overcome challenges and setbacks.

kids who have a growth mindset are more likely to take on new challenges and persist through difficult tasks.

They are also more likely to seek out feedback and learn from their mistakes, which can help them develop new skills and improve their performance.

Building resilience is also important for kids because it helps them cope with stress and adversity.

When kids are resilient, they are better able to handle difficult situations and recover from setbacks. This can help them maintain their mental health and well-being.

Building resilience and a growth mindset is important for children's personal and academic development.

It helps them develop the skills they need to succeed in school and life and helps them cope with stress and adversity.

Parents can help build resilience and a growth mindset by encouraging kids to take risks and learn from their mistakes.

Parents can also help kids develop a positive attitude toward learning by praising effort and persistence rather than just achievement.

Encouraging learning and growth is an essential part of building good kids.

Parents can help their kids develop a love of learning by creating a positive learning environment, providing opportunities for learning outside of the classroom, and building resilience and a growth mindset.

By doing so, parents can help their kids develop the knowledge, skills, and attitudes they need to succeed in life.

# Chapter 5:

Fostering Emotional Intelligence
Emotional intelligence is the ability to recognize, understand, and manage one's own emotions, as well as the emotions of others.

Developing emotional intelligence is an important part of building good kids. Here are some strategies for fostering emotional intelligence in children:

Understanding Emotional Intelligence
Emotional intelligence involves a variety of skills, including self-awareness, self-regulation, empathy, and social skills. Self-awareness involves recognizing one's

own emotions and how they affect one's thoughts and behavior.

Self-regulation involves managing one's emotions and behavior in appropriate ways. Empathy involves understanding and responding to the emotions of others.

Social skills involve communicating effectively, cooperating with others, and resolving conflicts.

Strategies for Fostering Emotional Intelligence
There are many ways to foster emotional intelligence in children. Here are some effective strategies:

1. Model emotional intelligence: kids learn by watching their parents and other adults in their lives. Modeling emotional intelligence by expressing emotions in healthy ways, regulating emotions, and

showing empathy can help kids develop these skills.

For example, if a parent expresses their frustration calmly, the child may learn to do the same. If a parent shows empathy to someone in need, the child may learn to do the same.

2. Encourage emotional expression: Encouraging kids to express their emotions in healthy ways is important because it helps them to develop emotional intelligence.

Emotional intelligence is the ability to recognize and understand our own emotions, as well as the emotions of others. It involves being able to regulate our emotions healthily and to use our emotions to guide our thoughts and actions.

When kids are encouraged to express their emotions, they learn that it is safe to do so.

They learn that it is okay to feel sad, angry, or frustrated and that these feelings can be expressed in healthy ways. This can help kids to develop a sense of self-awareness, which is important for their emotional development.

Talking about their feelings is one way that kids can healthily express their emotions. When kids are encouraged to talk about their feelings, they learn to identify and label their emotions.

This can help them to understand their emotions better and to communicate their feelings to others.

When kids can communicate their feelings effectively, they are more likely to develop healthy relationships with others.

Engaging in creative activities like drawing or writing is another way that kids can healthily express their emotions.

When kids engage in creative activities, they can express their emotions in a non-verbal way.

This can be helpful for kids who have difficulty expressing their emotions through words.

Creative activities can also be a form of self-expression, which can help kids develop a sense of identity and self-esteem.

In addition to helping kids develop emotional intelligence, encouraging kids to express their emotions in healthy ways can also help them to regulate their emotions.

When kids can healthily express their emotions, they are less likely to engage in unhealthy behaviors like aggression or substance abuse.

They are also more likely to develop healthy coping strategies for dealing with difficult situations.

3. Teach emotional regulation: Helping kids learn to regulate their emotions by teaching them techniques such as deep breathing, mindfulness, or physical exercise is important because it can help kids healthily manage their emotions.

When kids learn to regulate their emotions, they are better able to cope with difficult situations, communicate effectively with others, and maintain healthy relationships.

Deep breathing is one technique that can help kids regulate their emotions.

When kids are feeling overwhelmed or anxious, taking deep breaths can help them to calm down and relax.

Deep breathing can also help kids to focus their attention, which can be helpful when they are feeling distracted or unfocused.

Mindfulness is another technique that can help kids to regulate their emotions.

Mindfulness involves paying attention to the present moment without judgment.

When kids practice mindfulness, they learn to observe their thoughts and feelings without getting caught up in them. This can help kids to develop a sense of calm and perspective, even in difficult situations.

Physical exercise is also an effective way to help kids regulate their emotions.

Exercise can help to release tension and stress and can also help to boost mood and energy levels.

When kids engage in physical activity, they are also more likely to feel a sense of accomplishment and self-esteem, which can be helpful for their emotional well-being.

4. Practice empathy: Encouraging kids to understand and respond to the emotions of others by practicing empathy is important because it helps kids develop strong social skills and build healthy relationships.

When the kids practice empathy, they learn to recognize and understand the emotions of others, and they are better able to respond with kindness and compassion.

Role-playing is one way to help kids practice empathy.

By pretending to be in someone else's shoes, kids can learn to see things from another person's perspective. This can help them to develop a deeper understanding of other people's feelings and needs.

Reading books about emotions is another effective way to help kids practice empathy.

By reading stories about different characters and their emotions, kids can learn to recognize and understand a wide range of feelings.

This can help them to develop empathy and compassion for others.

Discussing emotions in everyday situations is also an effective way to help kids practice empathy.

When kids learn to recognize and respond to emotions in everyday situations, they are better able to understand and empathize with others.

For example, when a friend is feeling sad, a kid can learn to respond with kindness and support.

5. Foster social skills: Helping kids develop social skills by teaching them effective communication, cooperation, and conflict resolution strategies is important because it can help them to build healthy relationships and succeed in social situations.

When kids learn social skills, they are better able to communicate effectively with others, work collaboratively in groups, and constructively resolve conflicts.

Effective communication is one important social skill that kids need to learn.

When kids learn to communicate effectively, they are better able to express their thoughts and feelings, listen to others, and build positive relationships.

Effective communication involves using clear language, active listening, and nonverbal communication.

Cooperation is another important social skill that kids need to learn.

When kids learn to cooperate, they are better able to work together with others to achieve common goals. Cooperation involves sharing, taking turns, and compromising.

Conflict resolution is also an important social skill that kids need to learn.

When kids learn to resolve conflicts constructively, they are better able to maintain healthy relationships and avoid negative outcomes.

Conflict resolution involves identifying the problem, listening to others, brainstorming solutions, and compromising.

Helping kid Manage Their Emotions
Managing emotions is an important part of emotional intelligence. Here are some tips for helping kids manage their emotions:

1. Validate their emotions: It is important to let kids know that it's okay to feel a wide range of emotions and that all emotions are valid because it can help them to develop a healthy relationship with their emotions.

When kids learn that all emotions are valid, they are better able to recognize and express their feelings, and they are less likely to suppress or deny their emotions.

Emotions are a natural and normal part of life, and all emotions serve a purpose.

When kids learn that it's okay to feel a wide range of emotions, they are better able to cope with the ups and downs of life.

They are also more likely to develop empathy and compassion for others as they learn to recognize and understand the emotions of others.

One way to let kids know that all emotions are valid is to encourage them to express their feelings freely.

When kids are allowed to express their emotions without judgment or criticism, they are more likely to develop a healthy relationship with their emotions.

This can involve creating a safe and supportive environment where kids feel comfortable sharing their feelings.

Another way to let kids know that all emotions are valid is to help them to recognize and name their emotions.

When kids learn to identify their emotions, they are better able to understand the causes of their feelings and healthily respond to them.

This can involve teaching kids to use "I" statements to express their feelings or helping them to identify the physical sensations associated with different emotions.

2. Teach coping strategies: It's important to help kids learn coping strategies for managing difficult emotions, such as taking a break, talking to someone, or engaging in a relaxing activity, because it can help them to regulate their emotions and healthily cope with stress.

When kids learn coping strategies, they are better able to manage their emotions, reduce their stress levels, and maintain their overall well-being.

Managing difficult emotions can be challenging for children, especially if they are not sure how to recognize or express their feelings.

By teaching kids coping strategies, we can help them to develop the skills they need to manage their emotions healthily.

Coping strategies can include physical activities, such as exercise or yoga, as well as mental activities, such as mindfulness or meditation.

One way to help kids learn coping strategies is to model healthy coping behaviors.

When kids see adults healthily managing their emotions, they are more likely to adopt these behaviors themselves.

This can involve taking breaks when feeling overwhelmed, engaging in self-care activities, and seeking support from others when needed.

Another way to help kids learn coping strategies is to provide them with a range of options for managing their emotions.

This can involve teaching kids relaxation techniques, such as deep breathing or visualization, as well as encouraging them to engage in physical activities, such as sports or dance.

It can also involve providing kids with opportunities to talk to a trusted adult or counselor about their feelings.

3. Encourage problem-solving: Parents need
to teach kids problem-solving strategies for
dealing with difficult situations that may
trigger strong emotions because it can help
kids to learn how to navigate challenges
healthily and productively.

When kids learn problem-solving strategies,
they are better equipped to manage their
emotions and respond to difficult situations
in a way that promotes their overall
well-being.

Kids can face a range of challenges that may
trigger strong emotions, such as conflicts
with peers, academic stress, or family issues.

By teaching kids problem-solving strategies,
parents can help them to develop the skills
they need to manage these challenges
healthily.

Problem-solving strategies can include
identifying the problem, brainstorming

solutions, evaluating the pros and cons of each solution, and selecting the best option.

One way to teach kids problem-solving strategies is to model healthy problem-solving behaviors.

When kids see adults using problem-solving strategies in their daily lives, they are more likely to adopt these behaviors themselves.

This can involve talking through problems with children, encouraging them to brainstorm solutions, and helping them to evaluate the pros and cons of different options.

Another way to teach kids problem-solving strategies is to provide them with opportunities to practice these skills.

This can involve role-playing scenarios with children, such as conflicts with peers or challenging academic assignments, and encouraging them to use problem-solving strategies to navigate these situations.

It can also involve providing kids with tools and resources, such as books or online resources, that can help them to develop their problem-solving skills.

By fostering emotional intelligence in children, parents and caregivers can help build good kids who are better equipped to manage their emotions, communicate effectively, and build healthy relationships.

# Chapter 6:

Promoting Health and Well-Being

Promoting health and well-being is an important part of building good kids.

Here are some strategies for promoting health and well-being in children:

The Importance of Health and Well-Being Health and well-being are critical for children's physical, mental, and emotional development.

Kids who are healthy and well-nourished are more likely to thrive and reach their full potential. Promoting health and well-being also helps prevent chronic diseases and other health problems later in life.

Strategies for Promoting Health and Well-Being

There are many ways to promote health and well-being in children. Here are some effective strategies:

1. Encourage physical activity: Regular physical activity is essential for children's health and well-being.

It's important to encourage kids to engage in at least 60 minutes of physical activity each day because physical activity is essential for children's physical, emotional, and social development.

Regular physical activity can help kids to build strong bones and muscles, maintain a healthy weight, and reduce their risk of developing chronic diseases later in life.

It can also help to improve children's mood, reduce their stress levels, and promote healthy social interactions with peers.

Physical activity is essential for children's physical development because it helps to build strong bones and muscles.

When kids engage in physical activity, such as running, jumping, or playing sports, their bodies are challenged in ways that promote the growth and development of their bones and muscles.

This can help to reduce their risk of developing conditions such as osteoporosis or sarcopenia later in life.

Physical activity is also important for children's emotional development because it can help to improve their mood and reduce their stress levels.

When kids engage in physical activity, their bodies release endorphins, which can help to improve their mood and reduce feelings of stress or anxiety.

Regular physical activity can also help to improve children's self-esteem and confidence, which can have a positive impact on their overall emotional well-being.

Finally, physical activity is important for children's social development because it can promote healthy social interactions with peers.

When kids engage in physical activity together, such as playing sports or riding bikes, they have the opportunity to develop important social skills, such as teamwork, communication, and sportsmanship.

These skills can help to promote positive relationships with peers and contribute to children's overall social development.

2. Provide healthy food choices: A healthy diet is essential for children's growth and development.

It's important to provide kids with a variety of healthy food choices, such as fruits, vegetables, whole grains, and lean proteins, because a healthy and balanced diet is essential for children's growth and development.

A diet that includes a variety of healthy foods can help kids to maintain a healthy weight, reduce their risk of developing chronic diseases later in life, and support their overall health and well-being.

When kids eat a variety of healthy foods, they are more likely to get the nutrients they need for healthy growth and development.

Fruits and vegetables are good sources of vitamins, minerals, and fiber, which are essential for healthy growth and development.

Whole grains provide energy and are a good source of fiber, while lean proteins, such as chicken, fish, and beans, provide essential amino acids for building and repairing tissues.

In addition to providing essential nutrients, a healthy and balanced diet can help kids to maintain a healthy weight.

By providing kids with healthy food choices, parents can help to promote healthy eating habits and prevent unhealthy weight gain. This can help to reduce children's risk of developing chronic diseases later in life, such as diabetes, heart disease, and certain types of cancer.

Finally, a healthy and balanced diet can support children's overall health and well-being.

By providing kids with healthy food choices, parents can help to support their immune systems, reduce their risk of developing infections, and promote healthy digestion.

A healthy diet can also help to improve children's mood and reduce their risk of developing mental health problems, such as depression and anxiety.

3. Promote good sleep habits: Adequate sleep is critical for children's physical and mental health. Encouraging kids to establish consistent sleep routines and get the recommended amount of sleep each night is important for their overall health and well-being.

Getting enough sleep is essential for children's growth and development, and it can have a significant impact on their physical and mental health.

When kids get enough sleep, it can help to support their physical growth and development.

During sleep, the body releases growth
hormones that are essential for healthy
growth and development. Kids who get
enough sleep are more likely to reach their
full growth potential and have a healthy
weight.

Sleep is also important for children's mental
health. Kids who get enough sleep are more
likely to have better mental health,
including improved mood, behavior, and
cognitive function.

They are also less likely to experience
problems with attention, learning, and
memory.

Establishing consistent sleep routines can
help kids get enough sleep each night. This
includes setting a regular bedtime and
wake-up time, creating a calming bedtime
routine, and avoiding stimulating activities
before bed, such as screen time.

By establishing consistent sleep routines, parents can help to promote healthy sleep habits and improve their children's overall health and well-being.

4. Teach stress management skills: Stress can have negative effects on children's health and well-being.

Teaching kids stress management skills, such as deep breathing, mindfulness, or physical activity, is important for their mental and physical health.

Stress is a normal part of life, but too much stress can have negative effects on children's health and well-being.

Stress can cause physical symptoms, such as headaches, stomachaches, and muscle tension.

It can also cause mental and emotional symptoms, such as anxiety, depression, and irritability.

When kids learn stress management skills, they can better cope with stress and reduce the negative effects it has on their health.

Deep breathing is a simple and effective stress management technique that can be used anywhere, anytime.

It involves taking slow, deep breaths in through the nose and out through the mouth. This can help to slow the heart rate, lower blood pressure, and reduce feelings of stress and anxiety.

Mindfulness is another stress management technique that involves being present at the moment and focusing on the present experience.

This can help to reduce stress and anxiety by promoting relaxation and reducing negative thoughts and emotions.

Physical activity is also an effective stress management technique that can help to reduce stress and improve overall health and well-being.

Exercise releases endorphins, which are natural mood boosters that can help to reduce feelings of stress and anxiety.

5. Encourage positive social interactions: Positive social interactions are important for children's emotional well-being.

Encouraging kids to build positive relationships with peers and adults, and to engage in activities that promote social connectedness, is important for their social and emotional development.

Positive relationships and social connections have been linked to better mental health, increased self-esteem, and improved academic performance.

Building positive relationships with peers and adults can help kids to feel supported, valued, and connected to their community.

This can have a positive impact on their mental health and well-being, as well as their academic performance.

Kids who feel connected to their community are more likely to have positive attitudes toward school and learning and are more likely to succeed academically.

Engaging in activities that promote social connectedness, such as team sports, clubs, or community service, can also help kids to build positive relationships and develop important social skills.

These activities provide kids with opportunities to interact with others in a positive and supportive environment and to develop important skills such as communication, teamwork, and leadership.

Building Healthy Habits
Building healthy habits is an important part of promoting health and well-being in children. Here are some tips for building healthy habits:

1. Start early: Establish healthy habits early in life to help kids develop lifelong healthy behaviors.

2. Make it fun: Engage kids in fun activities that promote physical activity and healthy eating, such as cooking healthy meals together or playing active games.

3. Involve the whole family: Encourage the whole family to engage in healthy behaviors

together, such as going for walks or bike rides or preparing healthy meals together.

4. Be a role model: kids learn by watching their parents and other adults in their lives. Be a positive role model for healthy behaviors.

By promoting health and well-being in kids and building healthy habits early in life, parents and caregivers can help build good kids.

# Chapter 7:

Nurturing Relationships with Others

Nurturing relationships with others is an important part of building good kids. Here are some strategies for nurturing relationships in children:

The Importance of Relationships
Relationships are critical for children's emotional and social development.

Positive relationships with peers and adults can help children build self-esteem, develop social skills, and learn how to communicate effectively.

Nurturing relationships can also help children feel supported and loved.

Strategies for Nurturing Relationships with Others

There are many ways to nurture relationships with others. Here are some effective strategies:

1. Encourage communication: Communication is key to building positive relationships.

Encouraging children to communicate openly and honestly with others, and to listen actively when others are speaking, is very important because it helps them develop important social and emotional skills that will be valuable throughout their lives.

When children learn to communicate openly and honestly with others, they are more likely to develop healthy relationships with peers, family members, and other adults in their lives.

They are also more likely to develop a sense
of self-awareness and self-expression that
will be valuable throughout their lives.

In addition, when children learn to listen
actively when others are speaking, they are
more likely to develop empathy and
understanding for others.

They are also more likely to develop
important communication skills that will be
valuable in both personal and professional
settings.

2. Foster positive interactions: Positive
interactions with others can help build
strong relationships.

Encouraging children to engage in activities
that promote positive interactions, such as
playing games, working on projects
together, or volunteering in the community,
is important because it can help them
develop important social and emotional

skills that will be valuable throughout their lives.

When children engage in activities that promote positive interactions, they have the opportunity to develop important social skills such as teamwork, communication, and conflict resolution.

They also have the opportunity to develop important emotional skills such as empathy, compassion, and gratitude.

In addition, engaging in activities that promote positive interactions can help children develop a sense of community and belonging.

When children work together on a project or volunteer in the community, they have the opportunity to connect with others and develop a sense of purpose and meaning in their lives.

3. Teach conflict resolution skills: Conflict is a natural part of relationships.

Teaching children skills for resolving conflicts positively and respectfully, such as active listening, compromising, and finding common ground, is important because it can help them develop important social and emotional skills that will be valuable throughout their lives.

When children learn how to resolve conflicts positively and respectfully, they are more likely to develop healthy relationships with peers, family members, and other adults in their lives.

They are also more likely to develop a sense of self-awareness and self-control that will be valuable throughout their lives.

In addition, when children learn how to resolve conflicts positively and respectfully, they are more likely to develop empathy and understanding for others.

They are also more likely to develop important communication skills that will be valuable in both personal and professional settings.

4. Encourage empathy and compassion: Empathy and compassion are important for building positive relationships.

Encouraging children to consider others' feelings and perspectives, and to show kindness and compassion towards others, is important because it can help them develop important social and emotional skills that will be valuable throughout their lives.

When children learn how to consider others' feelings and perspectives, they are more likely to develop empathy and understanding for others. They are also more likely to develop important communication skills that will be valuable in both personal and professional settings.

In addition, when children learn how to show kindness and compassion towards others, they are more likely to develop healthy relationships with peers, family members, and other adults in their lives.

They are also more likely to develop a sense of self-awareness and self-control that will be valuable throughout their lives.

Teaching Empathy and Compassion
Teaching empathy and compassion is an important part of nurturing relationships with others. Here are some tips for teaching empathy and compassion:

1. Model empathy and compassion: Children learn by watching others, and as such, being a positive role model for empathy and compassion is important.

By showing kindness and understanding towards others, you can help children develop important social and emotional skills that will be valuable throughout their lives.

When children see positive examples of empathy and compassion, they are more likely to develop these skills themselves. They are also more likely to develop a sense of social responsibility and a desire to help others.

In addition, when children see positive examples of empathy and compassion, they are more likely to develop important social and emotional skills that will be valuable throughout their lives.

These skills include the ability to communicate effectively, the ability to understand and manage their emotions, and the ability to form healthy relationships with others.

# Chapter 8:

Raising Responsible and Independent kids.

Raising responsible and independent kids is an important part of building good kids, Here are some strategies for achieving this:

The Importance of Responsibility and Independence
Responsibility and independence are crucial for children's development. Kids who learn to take responsibility for their actions and become independent thinkers are more likely to succeed in school, work, and life in general.

They are also more likely to develop self-confidence and self-esteem.
Strategies for Raising Responsible and Independent Children.

Here are some strategies for raising responsible and independent children:

1. Give kids age-appropriate responsibilities:
Giving kids responsibilities helps them learn
how to take care of themselves and develop
independence.

Age-appropriate responsibilities can include
things like making their bed, cleaning up
their toys, and helping with household
chores.

2. Encourage decision-making: Encouraging
kids to make decisions helps them develop
critical thinking skills and independence.

Giving kids choices whenever possible, and
encouraging them to think through the pros
and cons of each option, is important
because it can help them develop important
decision-making skills that will be valuable
throughout their lives.

When kids are given choices, they are more
likely to develop a sense of autonomy and
independence.

They are also more likely to develop important problem-solving skills that will be valuable in both personal and professional settings.

In addition, when kids are encouraged to think through the pros and cons of each option, they are more likely to develop critical thinking skills that will be valuable throughout their lives.

They are also more likely to develop a sense of self-awareness and self-control that will be valuable throughout their lives.

3. Provide opportunities for problem-solving: Problem-solving is an important part of responsibility and independence.

Encouraging kids to solve problems on their own, and providing guidance and support when needed, is important because it can help them develop important problem-solving skills that will be valuable throughout their lives.

When kids are encouraged to solve problems on their own, they are more likely to develop a sense of autonomy and independence.

They are also more likely to develop important critical thinking skills that will be valuable in both personal and professional settings.

In addition, when kids are provided with guidance and support when needed, they are more likely to develop a sense of self-awareness and self-control that will be valuable throughout their lives.

They are also more likely to develop a sense of resilience and perseverance that will be valuable throughout their lives.

4. Set clear expectations: Setting clear expectations helps kids understand what is expected of them and encourages responsibility because it provides them with a framework for their behavior.

When kids know what is expected of them, they are more likely to behave in a way that meets those expectations.

This can lead to a sense of responsibility and accountability for their actions.

Clear expectations also provide kids with a sense of structure and routine, which can be comforting and reassuring.

When kids know what to expect, they are less likely to feel anxious or uncertain about their environment. This can help them feel more secure and confident in their abilities.

In addition, setting clear expectations can help kids develop self-discipline and self-control.

When kids know what is expected of them, they can learn to regulate their behavior and make choices that align with those expectations.

This can help them develop a sense of personal responsibility and self-efficacy. Be clear about what you expect from your children, and follow through with consequences when expectations are not met.

Encouraging Autonomy and Decision-Making
Encouraging autonomy and decision-making is an important part of raising responsible and independent children.

Here are some tips for encouraging autonomy and decision-making:

1. Let kids make mistakes: It's important to let kids make mistakes and learn from them, rather than trying to protect them from failure, because making mistakes is an important part of the learning process.

When kids make mistakes, they have the opportunity to learn from their experiences and develop important problem-solving skills.

If parents or caregivers try to protect kids from failure, they may inadvertently prevent them from developing important skills and abilities.

Kids who are shielded from failure may not develop the resilience and perseverance they need to overcome challenges and succeed in life.

In addition, letting kids make mistakes can help them develop a sense of autonomy and independence.

When kids are allowed to make their own decisions and experience the consequences of those decisions, they are more likely to develop a sense of responsibility and self-reliance.

Of course, it's important to provide support and guidance when kids make mistakes. Parents or caregivers can help kids reflect on their experiences and identify what they can learn from them.

This can help kids develop the skills they need to navigate challenges and overcome obstacles in the future.

2. Encourage risk-taking: Encouraging kids to take risks helps them develop confidence and independence because it helps them learn to trust their abilities and judgment.

When kids take risks, they learn to face challenges with courage and resilience. This can help them develop a sense of confidence in their abilities and a belief in their capacity to succeed.

Taking risks also helps kids develop a sense of independence. When kids take risks, they learn to make decisions and take action on their own.

This can help them develop a sense of autonomy and self-reliance, which can be important for their future success.

Encouraging kids to take risks can also help them develop problem-solving skills. When kids take risks, they learn to think creatively and develop solutions to problems.

This can help them develop critical thinking skills and learn to approach challenges with a positive and proactive mindset.

3. Provide guidance and support: While it's important to encourage autonomy and decision-making, kids still need guidance and support because they are still developing their decision-making abilities and may not have the experience or knowledge to make the best decisions on their own.

Guidance and support can come in many forms, such as providing information, offering advice, or setting boundaries.

When parents or caregivers provide guidance and support, they can help kids make informed decisions and avoid potential risks or negative consequences. Guidance and support can also help kids develop a sense of trust and security.

When kids know that they can turn to their parents or caregivers for guidance and support, they are more likely to feel safe and secure in their environment.

This can help them develop a sense of confidence and resilience that will be valuable throughout their lives.

In addition, guidance and support can help kids develop important social and emotional skills, such as empathy, communication, and problem-solving.

When parents or caregivers provide guidance and support, they can model positive behaviors and help kids develop the skills they need to navigate social situations and build healthy relationships.

4. Celebrate successes: Celebrating successes, no matter how small, helps kids develop self-confidence and self-esteem because it helps them feel valued and recognized for their efforts.

When kids receive positive feedback for their accomplishments, they are more likely to feel proud of themselves and develop a sense of confidence in their abilities.

Celebrating successes can also help kids develop a growth mindset. When kids receive positive feedback for their accomplishments, they are more likely to view challenges as opportunities for growth and learning.

This can help them develop a sense of resilience and perseverance that will be valuable throughout their lives.

In addition, celebrating successes can help kids develop a sense of belonging and connection.

When kids receive positive feedback for their accomplishments, they are more likely to feel connected to their family, friends, and community.

This can help them develop a sense of social and emotional well-being that will be valuable throughout their lives.

By following these strategies and encouraging autonomy and decision-making, parents and caregivers can help raise responsible and independent kids who are confident, self-reliant, and successful.

## Conclusion

As parents, it's important to remember that raising good kids is a long-term process that requires patience, consistency, and perseverance. By applying the strategies outlined in this book, you can help your child develop into a well-rounded and successful individual.

Remember, you're not alone on this journey. Seek support from family, friends, or professionals when needed. Don't be afraid to ask for help or advice when you need it.

I hope that this book has been helpful and informative for you as a parent or caregiver. By working together, we can raise a generation of good kids who will make the world a better place.

www.ingramcontent.com/pod-product-compliance
Lightning Source LLC
Chambersburg PA
CBHW070912260726

48661CB00004B/1703